I Love You From My Head Tomatoes

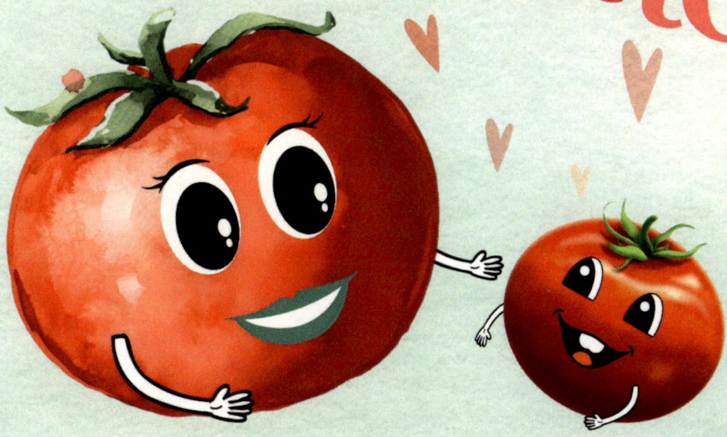

By Jerry Lott
Pictures by BRAINYINK

I Love You From My Head Tomatoes

By Jerry Lott

ISBN: 978-1-7637782-7-6
Publisher: BigStar Publishing

For more information, address: Sinjressforall@gmail.com.

This book is dedicated to all awesome kids

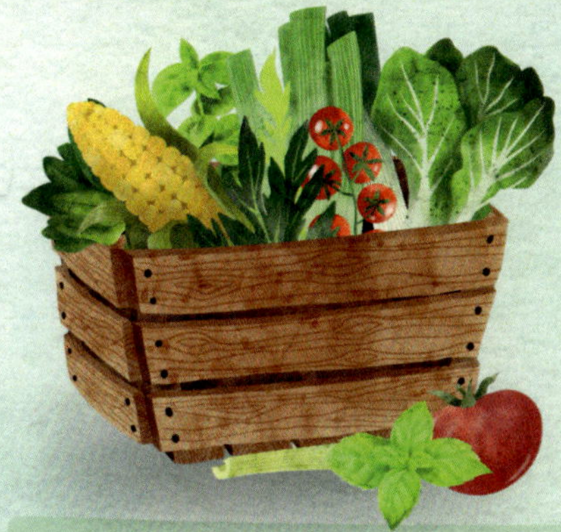

I utterly love you from my head
To-ma-toes,
Right down to my roots where
true love grows.

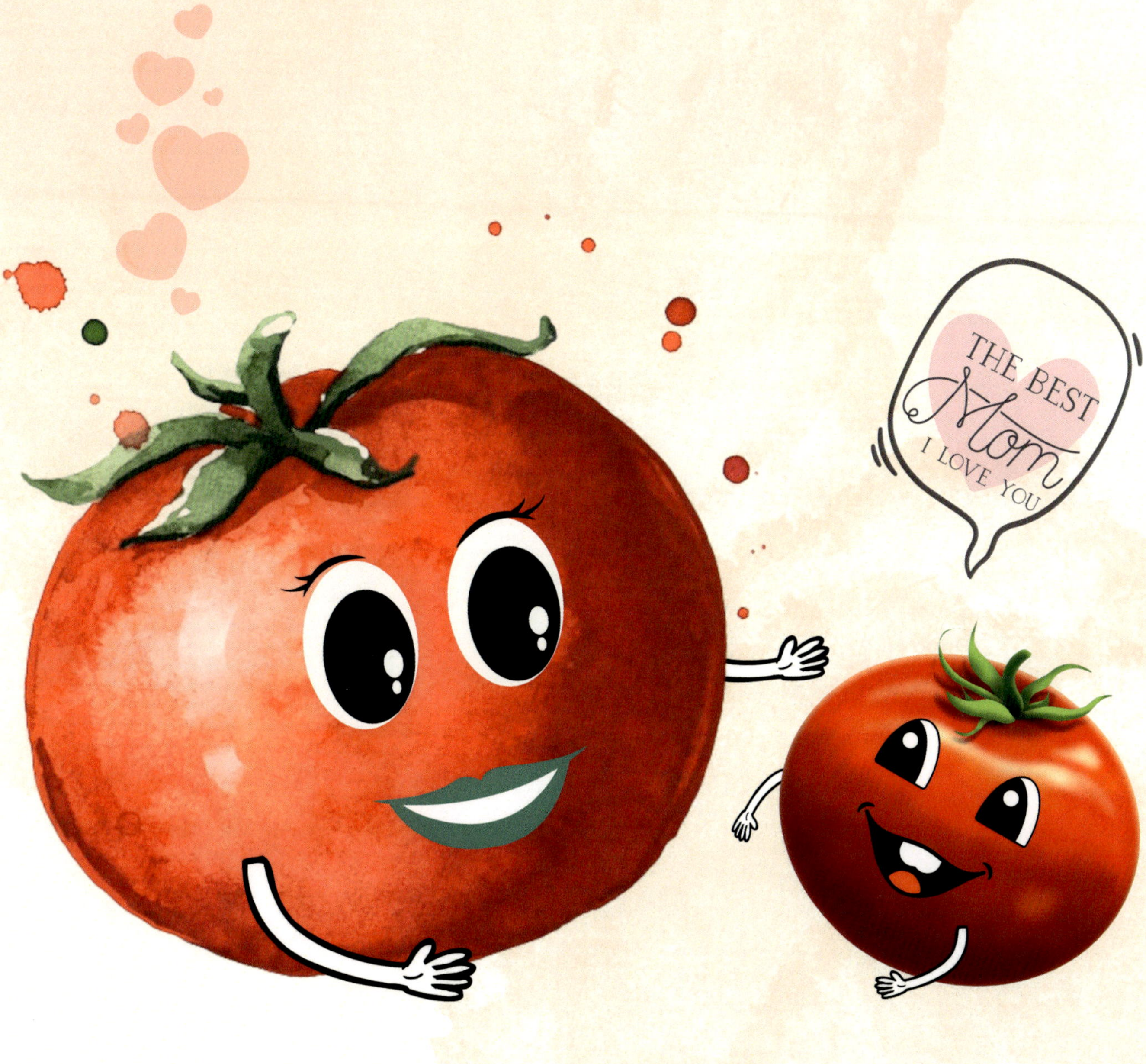
THE BEST
Mom
I LOVE YOU

Peas believe you're my
sweetest pea,
A precious and perfect pod
for all to see.

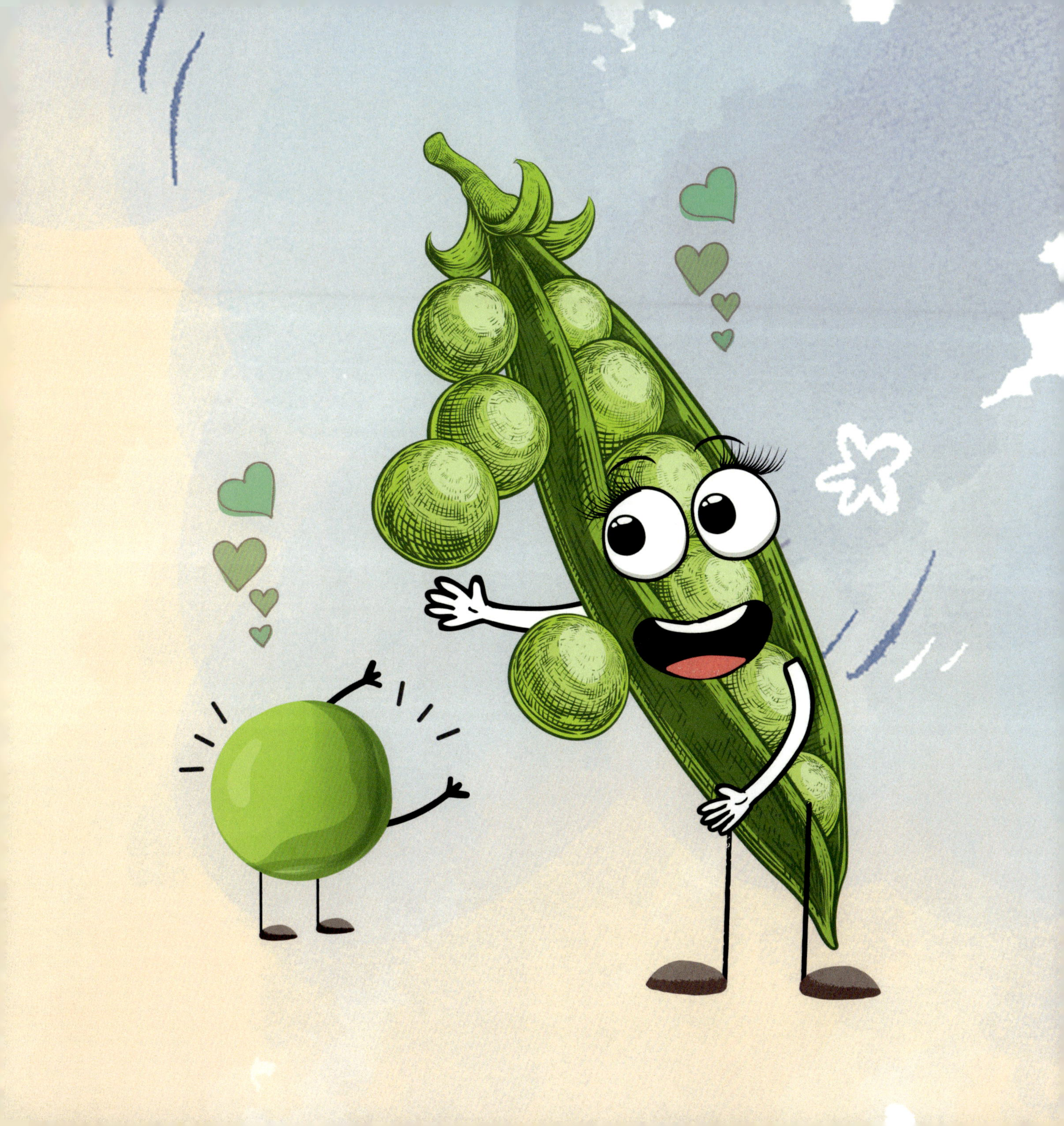

I **Carrot** help but love you so and so,

No matter what you do, no matter where you go.

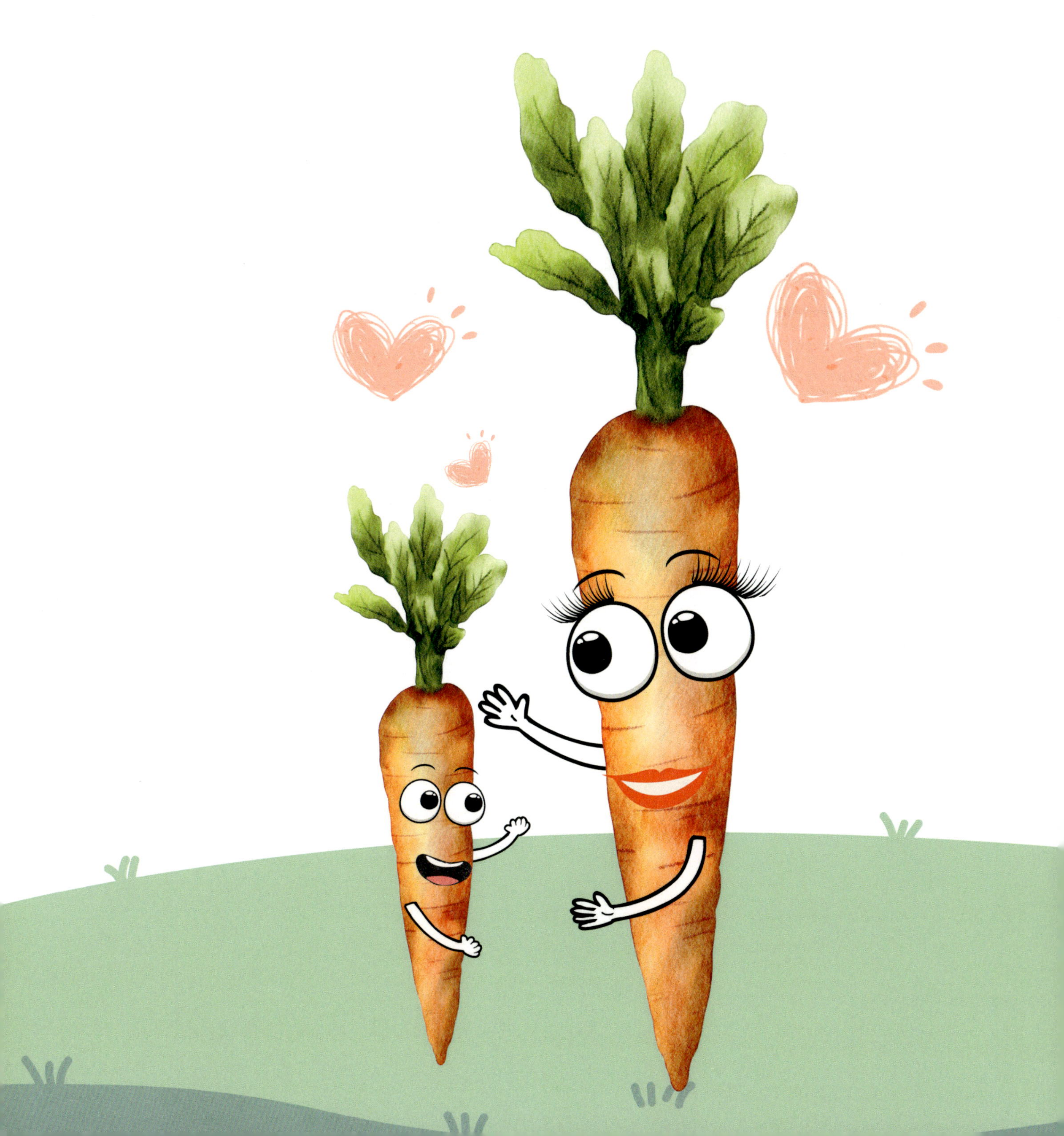

You make my heart sing and
skip every **Beet** ,
Your love, baby, is the
sweetest treat!

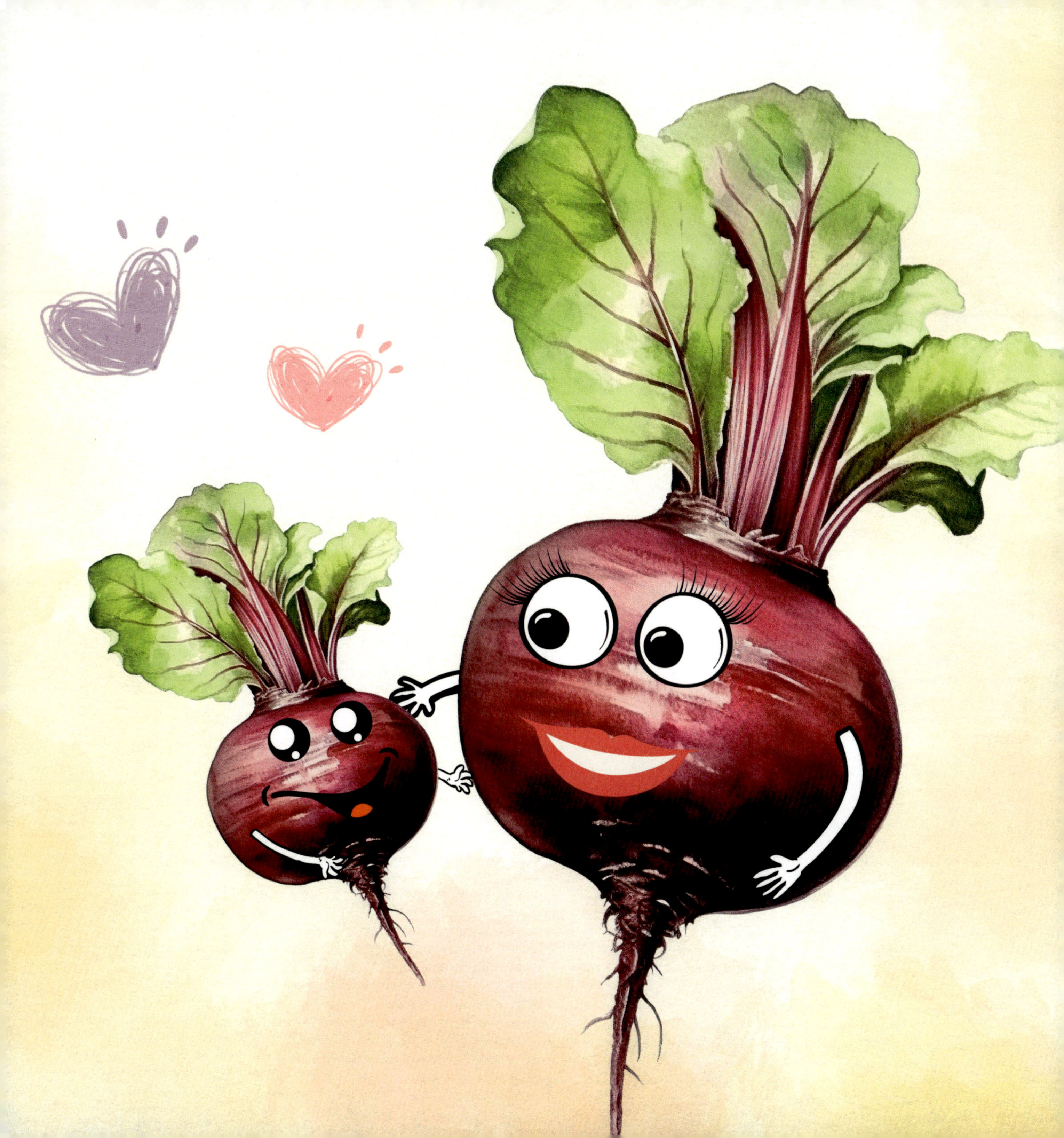

You're my little **sprout**, so
bright and true,
I'm forever **root**-ing for
everything you do.

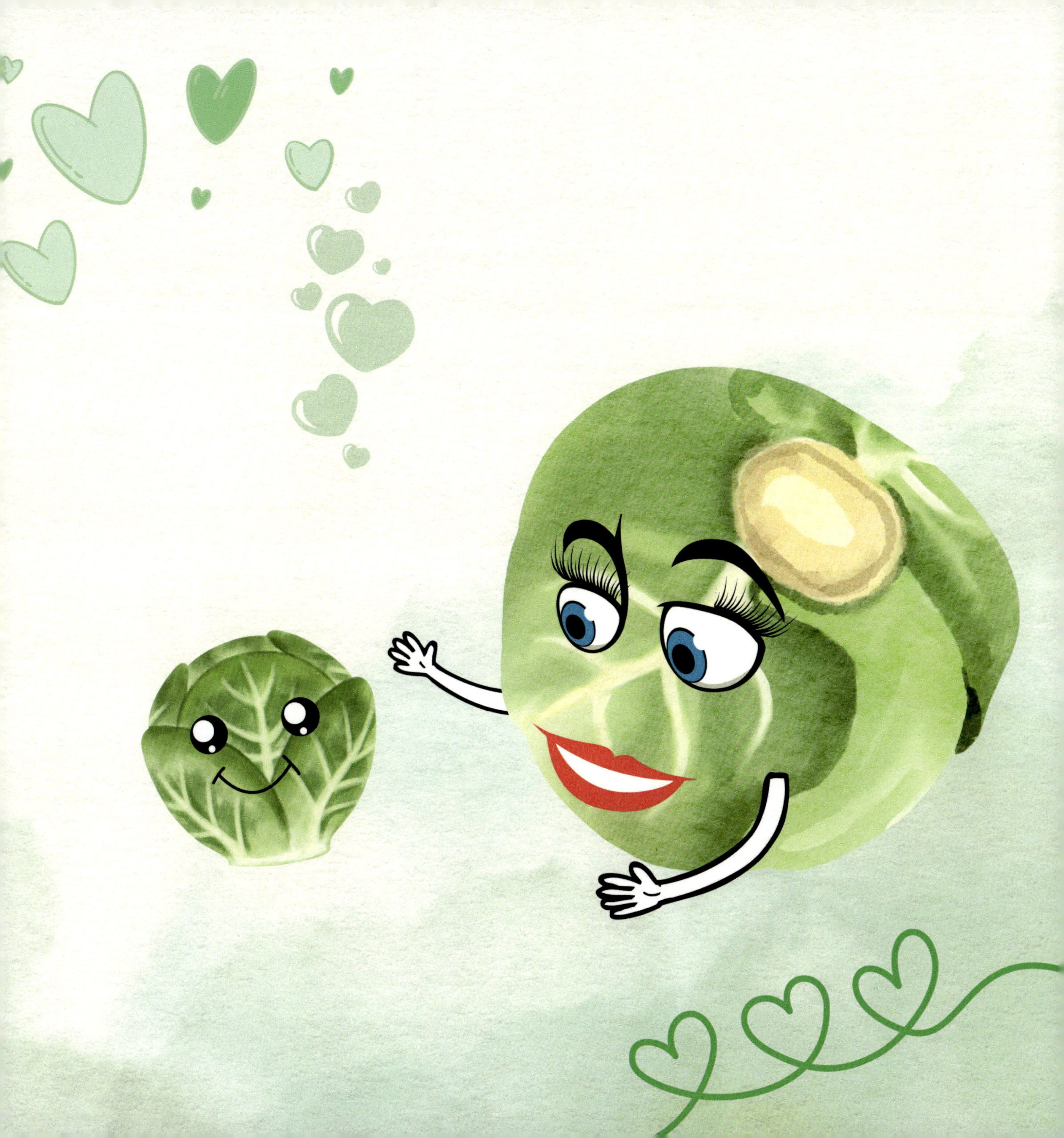

You're my **spud** -tacular
shooting star,
My pride, my joy, my love, just
as you are.

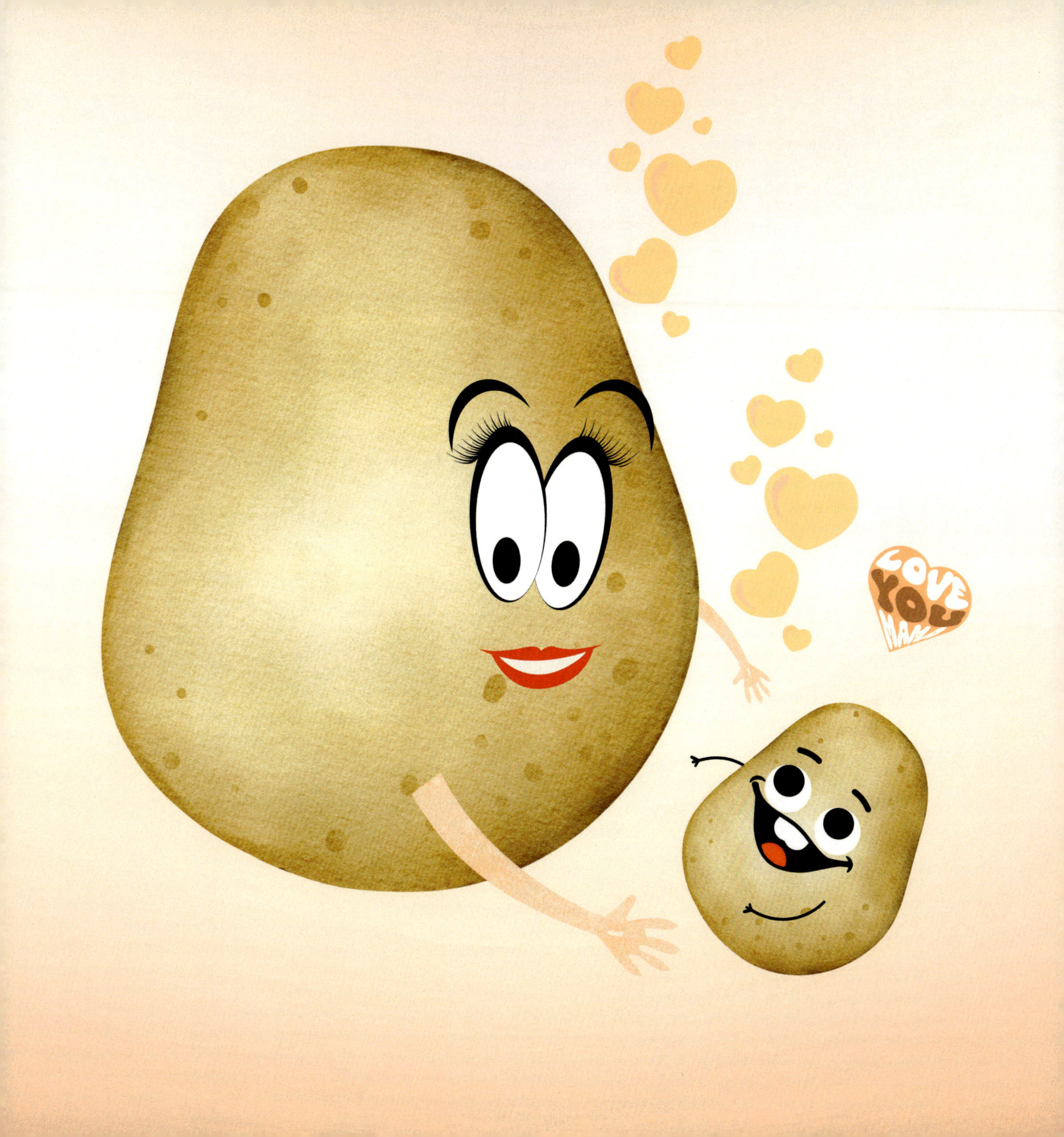
LOVE
YOU
MAM

lettuce forever remain side by side,
Always together, with love our shining guide.

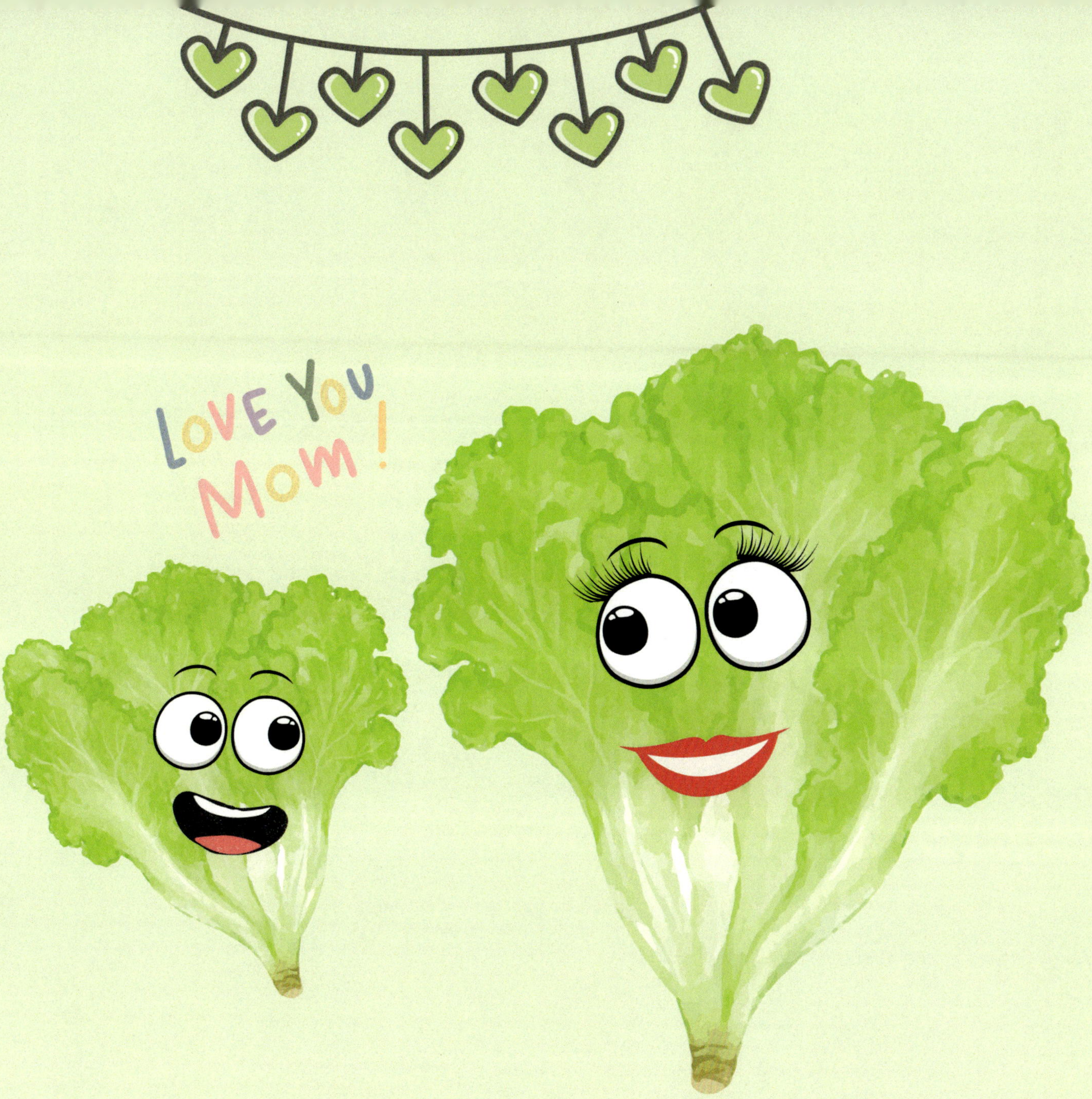
Love You
Mom!

You're **radishing** , my love, in every single way,
You turn up the charm each and every day.

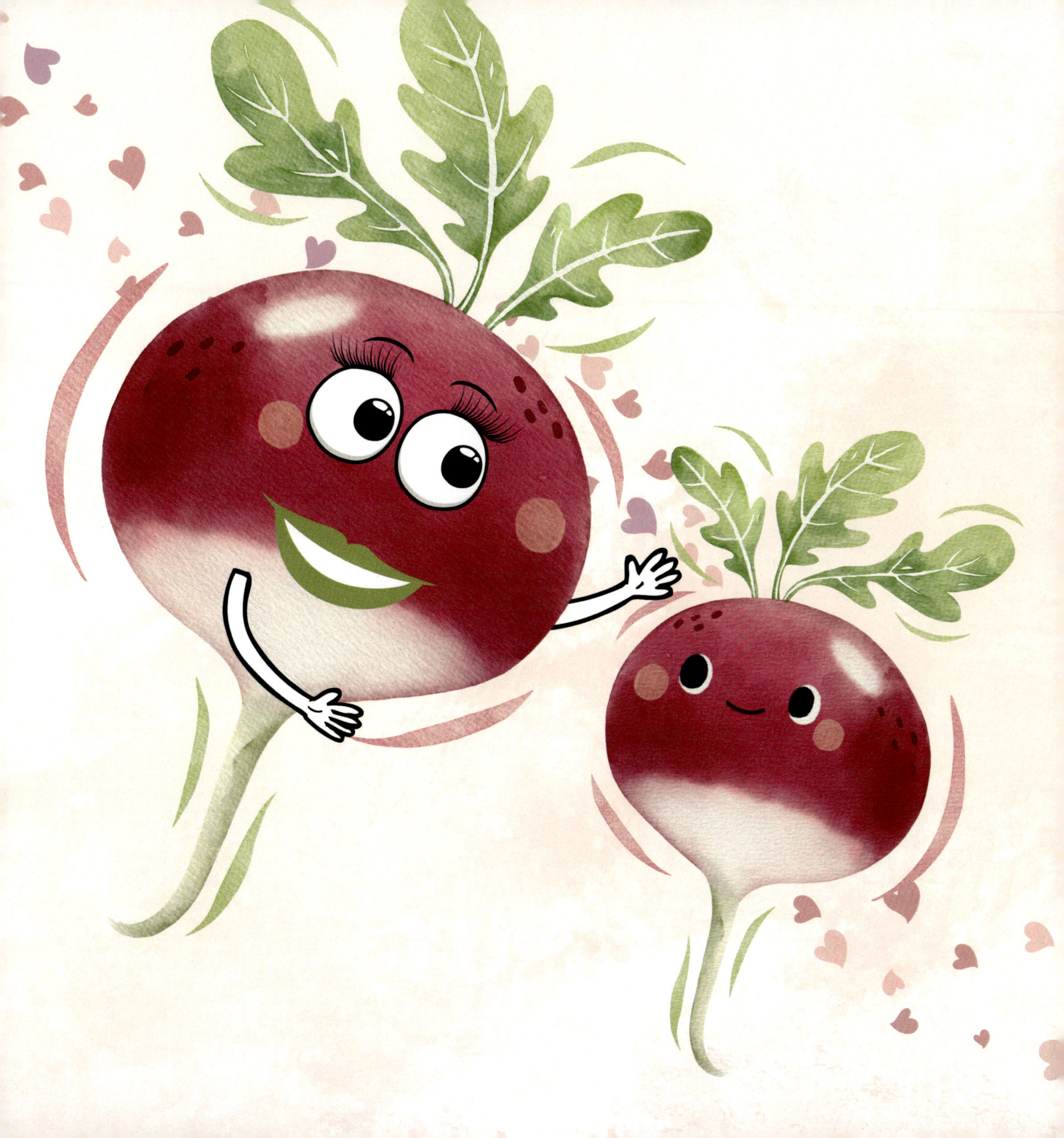

You've **bean** my joy and
sheer since day one,
Your love brightens my life,
my shining sun.

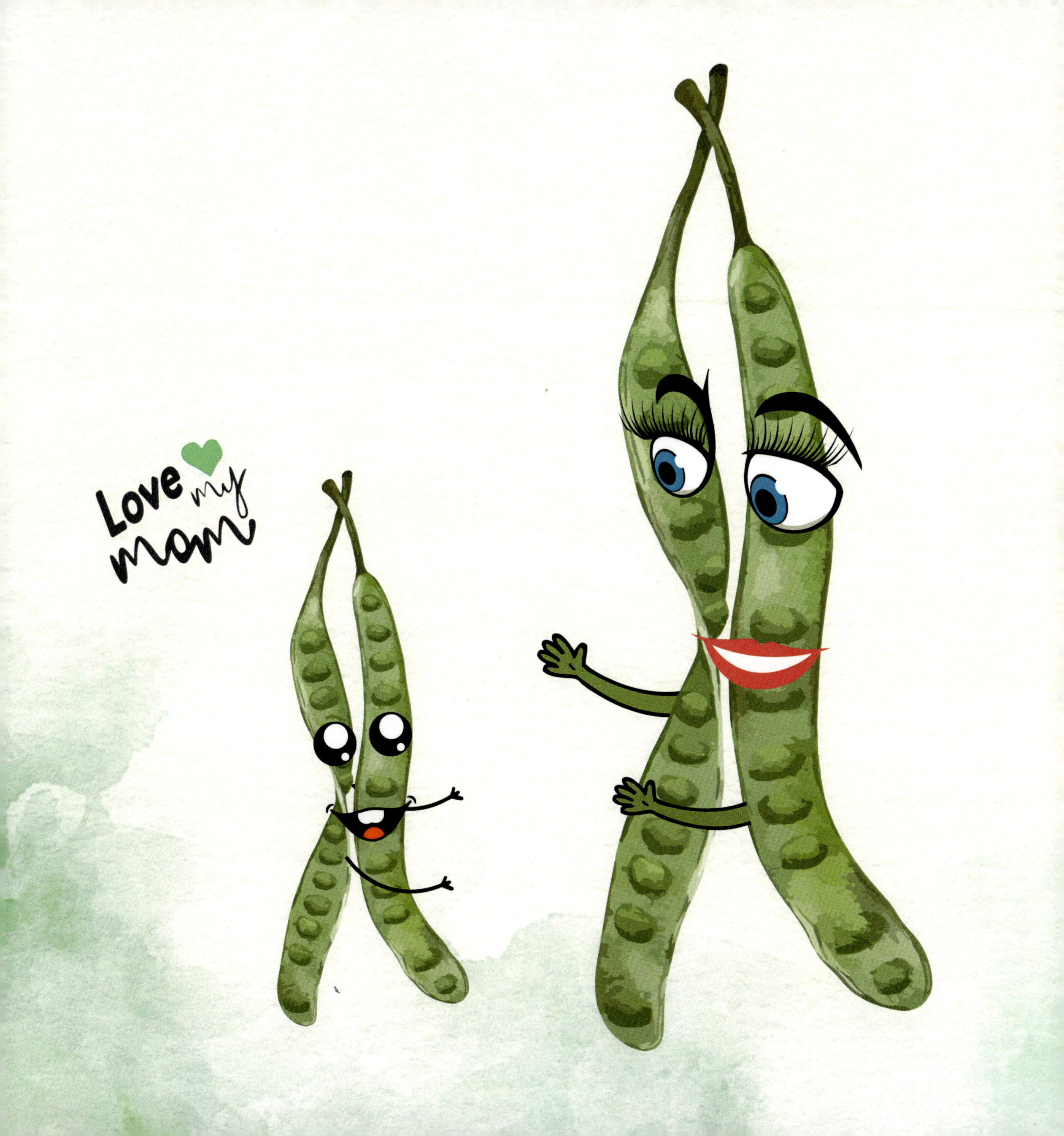
Love my mom

Every **thyme** we're together, love's in the room, You light up my life and fill it with bloom

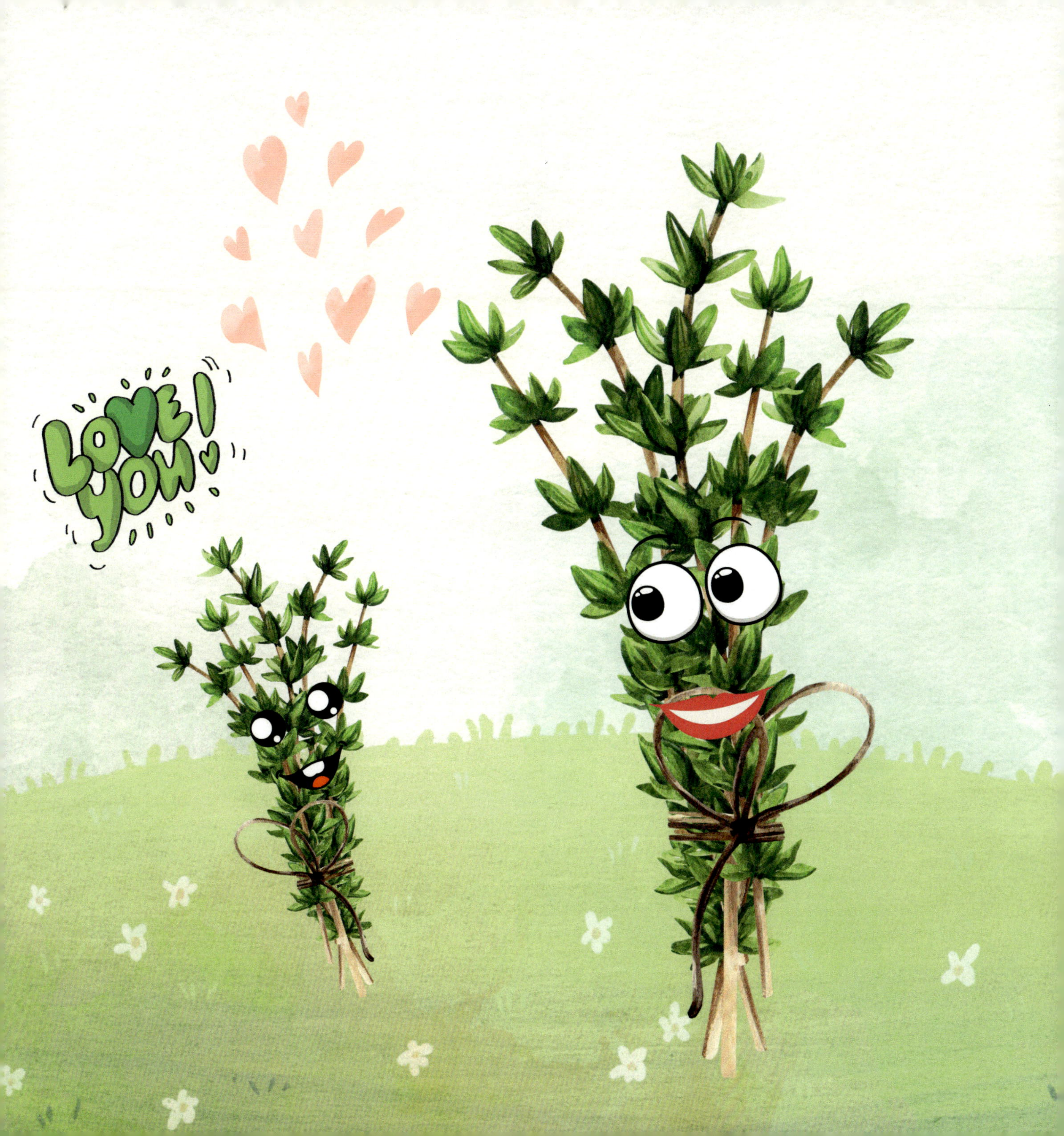
LOVE YOU!

I love you **onion** and on,
today and tomorrow
You bring tears of joy, never
of sorrow

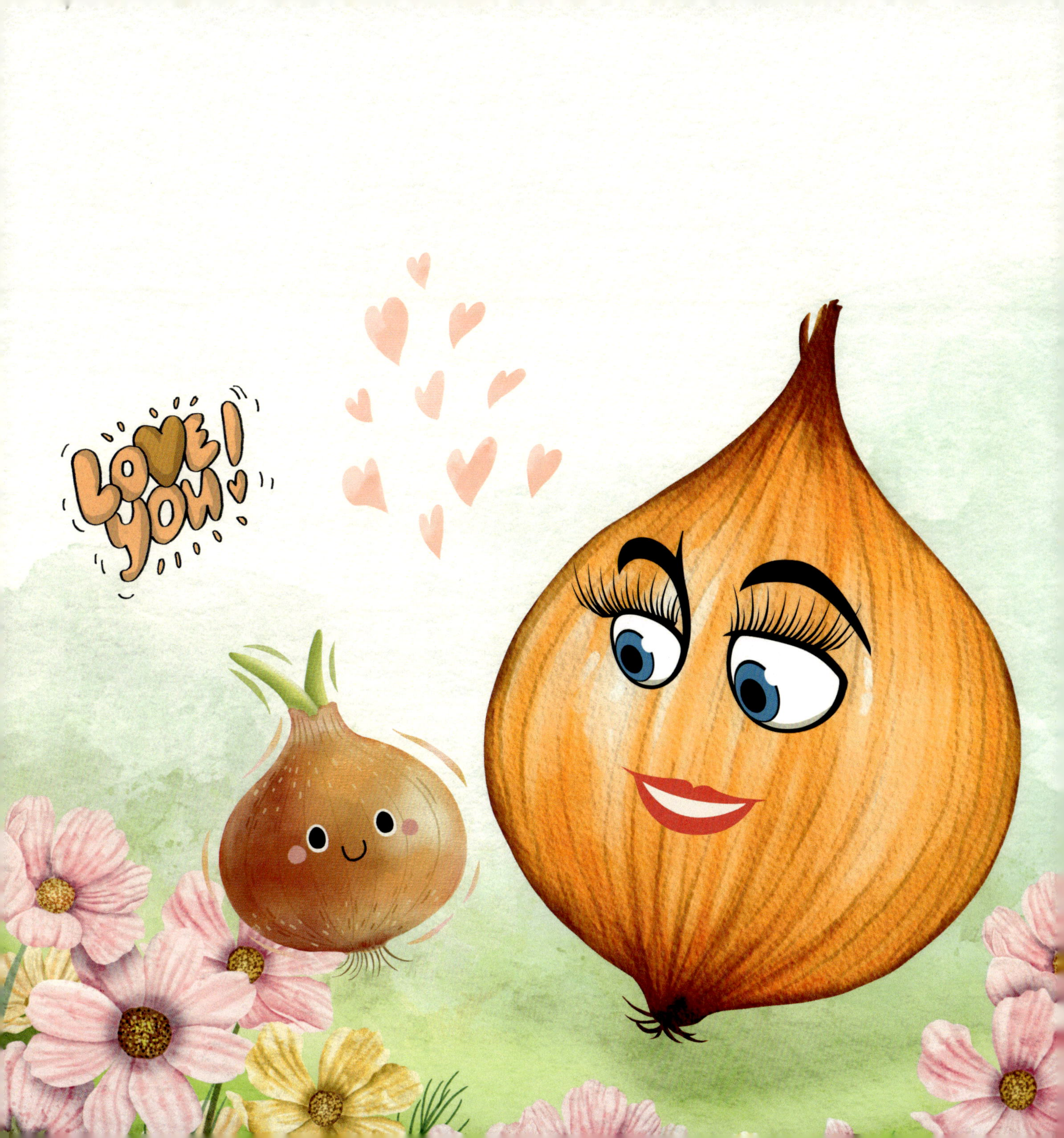
LOVE YOU!

I have so **mush-room** for
you in my heart
Come what may, we'll never
be apart

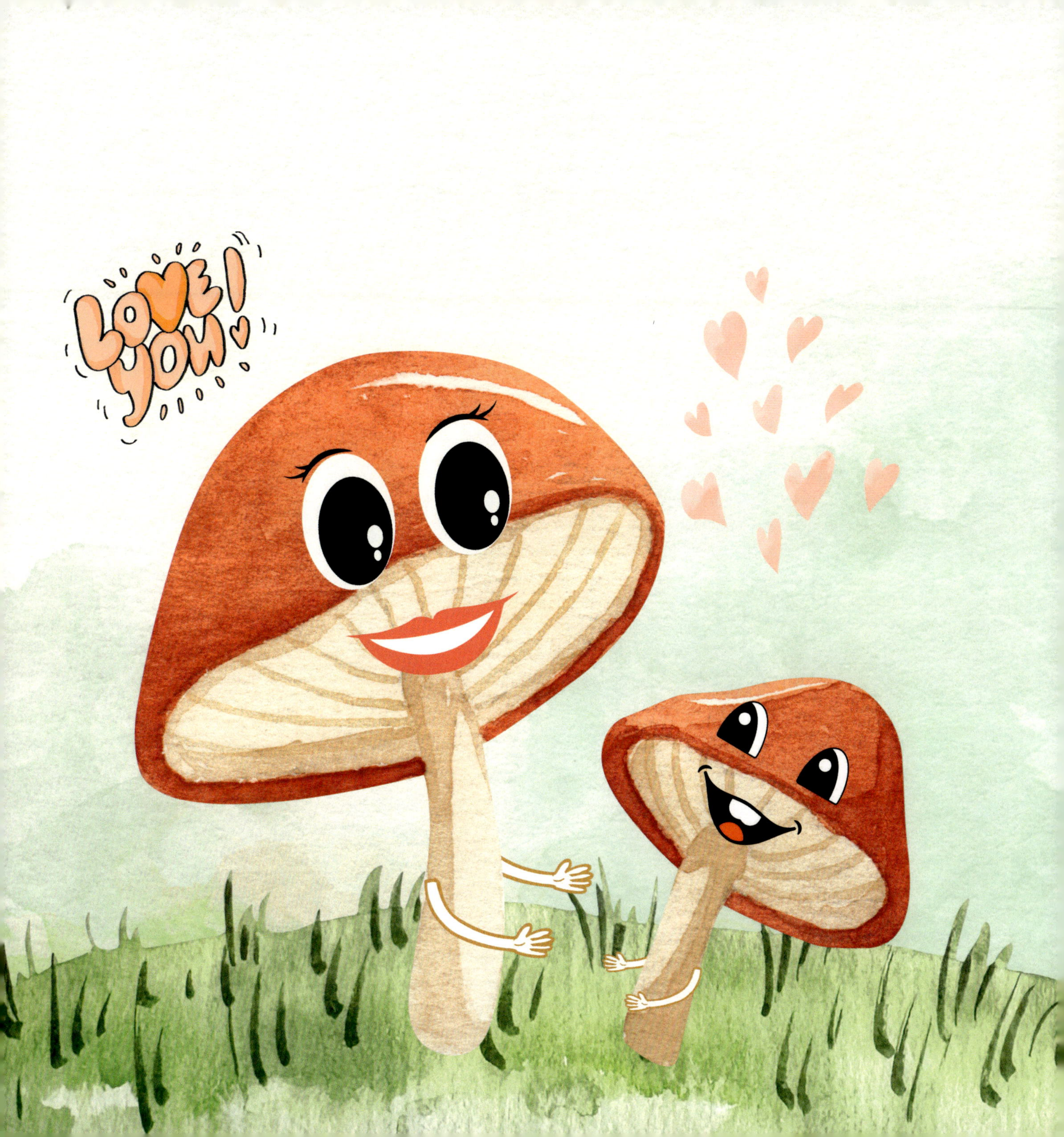
LOVE YOU!

Made in United States
Orlando, FL
26 June 2026

83335000R00017